EAT HEALTHY

LIVE LONGER, LOOK YOUNGER

ANTHONY EKANEM

ISBN 978-1-63997-766-6

Contents

Preface

When it comes to eating, how many of us bother to check whether we are eating healthy food? The lifestyle of today is so busy and excited that you eat food that tastes good but tends to neglect its negative effect on your health. There are several reasons and benefits of healthy eating, and you should take time to prepare healthy foods and diets for healthy living.

Here are the benefits of healthy eating:

- Apart from feeling and looking good, your body will be high on energy and fresh. With healthy food, you will enjoy doing everything and live a full life. Healthy eating leads to a healthier life and you find little or no reason to visit a doctor. You can spend time in more physical activities to keep fit.

- A healthy diet keeps the immune system more potent, and health problems are kept far away. A healthy immune system will ensure that you stay fit, and if sick, you will recover fast

- Healthy diets help you stay in shape. A well-planned and nutritious food helps to maintain your weight, and you save yourself from the worry of losing or gaining weight.

- Your brain gets alert and sharp, which helps you to perform well in all your activities. Research has shown that healthy food helps the brain to think well even at old age. You must have seen old people who are fit and fine even in their 80s, and this can be attributable to healthy food intake.

- A wholesome diet gives you all the essential minerals and nutrients that fulfil all the needs of the body.

- A healthy diet has proved to keep humans in a happy mood. Therefore, you will enjoy every moment of life and stay calm in any situation.

- Your skin is the face of your body. And the secret of glowing skin is healthy food. This does not only make you look great, but you feel strengthened from within.

- A good diet is essential for growing children. Children are very active, burn a lot of calories, and thus require all the proteins, carbohydrates, fats, and nutrients to stay fit.

- Healthy food keeps away many diseases and ill effects, and you will live a life that is free of tension and health problems. Apart from enjoying life, you will develop positive feelings. A healthy diet keeps both the mind and body fit.

It is not too late to start eating healthy food and so live a healthier life. It is always good to eat well and stay in good shape. You can keep overweight and other health problems far from you by eating healthy.

Why You Should Eat Healthy Food

The survival of the fittest is the principle that rules the animal kingdom. This rule does not apply to humankind, and as a result, they have consigned their health to the bottom of their priority list. It is only when nature delivers a dreadful reminder of negligence through a stroke, heart attack, or other serious health conditions that most people realise that they should have adopted a healthy lifestyle and routine.

The steps to follow to live a healthy life are very simple. Regular exercises and intake of the right kind of foods keep the body fit and develop a robust immune system to fight the onslaught of any disease. Eat the correct proportion of fats, proteins, and carbohydrates to provide the vitamins, minerals and other essential nutrients needed by the body to glow and flourish.

Carbohydrate-rich foods have a combination of fibre, sugar and starch, and thus supply the body with the glucose that provides the energy to complete physical tasks. Proteins are also important in providing energy to the body, but you must watch out for foods that have unhealthy amounts of fat and protein.

The right blend of fresh vegetables, fruits, dairy products, and meat can fulfil your body's daily nutritional needs. This means you can perform all the physical tasks as your brain remains healthy and active. A healthy body and mind do not only ensure a long and healthy life but also reduces common diseases drastically. It delays age-related illnesses, such as Alzheimer's or osteoporosis, therefore improving the quality of life.

Promote healthy eating habits among your family and loved ones. The right food helps you increase to be efficient while exercising and during physical work. A healthy mind can keep stress away, and this results in general wellbeing.

Eating unhealthy foods for a long period can lead to fat accumulation in different parts of the body, including the arteries. While body fat is visible, fat accumulating inside the body is not visible and it is unfortunately irreversible. If this happens, you might need to go for a heart bypass operation to replace any clogged arteries, if you are careless with your health for a long time. The key to enjoying your life is to embrace healthy eating habits. For girls and women, healthy eating habits will result in spotless skin and a fit body. The right combination of a heavy breakfast, medium lunch, and a light dinner can help the body to perform more efficiently.

As the old saying goes: 'prevention is better than cure'. And by eating healthy foods, you are on the road to living a long and healthy life. A healthy diet will enable you to perform all physical and mental functions optimally while ensuring that you live a better quality of life, free from many common ailments.

The Secrets to Eating Healthy

These days, people do not care to understand the importance of healthy eating. The consumption of junk foods has increased such that obesity and other health conditions are taking a heavy toll on their body. We all desire a flawless body and fresh-looking skin and face.

We have genuine desires to maintain our bodies, but the stress and anxieties of our daily lives have continued to hurt our bodies. The only remedy for this situation is to find a healthy balance by eating healthy foods. By taking extra time to prepare and eat good food, you will make your life fit and healthful.

Never leave your home without a wholesome breakfast. Always make some time in your schedule for eating. If you want to look good, you must eat well. Your meal must include the correct mix of salads, vegetables, and fruits. If you eat fruits after your meals, you will be high on energy and toxins will be removed from your body. If you are tending to overweight, avoid eating foods that contain saturated fats. Such foods will add to your body fat.

Eating healthy comprises avoiding too much alcohol, drugs, and other negative health habits. They would destroy your body cells and make you look pale and unattractive. In its place, get into the habit of taking fresh fruit juices daily. A glass of milk daily can also do wonders for your body. Avoid the temptation to eat meat every day. Instead, eat a vegetable dish. Your body needs a wholesome diet and depriving it would have serious health implications.

If you often complain of stress and body pains, you can blame it on your diet and eating habits. A healthy diet will keep you off stress and make you look great even at the end of a hectic day. Appropriate meals provide all the nutrients the body needs to stay fit and lively all day long. You would not need to visit a salon to get a glow on your face through artificial means. Nutritious foods take care of your health and beauty and give you a natural glow on your face. Your skin will look clear and clean, making you confident, and saving you from buying costly creams and skin products.

Always carry some healthy snacks when travelling. This prevents you from staying hungry. Fresh juice and fruits should be a good part of your stock. You should have 'no time to eat', as this is a very lame excuse. Just as you have time for your work, you should also have time to eat. All it requires is to set aside an eating schedule and stick to it. Eating should be your priority. When in a restaurant, make sure you order something healthy and strengthening.

Do not overeat as it will do you no good. Only eat when you are hungry. Do not be in the habit of changing your eating hours, otherwise, your body will suffer for it. If you have been a lot of junk food, it is time to start with healthy eating so you can live a more healthy life.

CHAPTER TWO

Recipes for Healthy Eating

Are you eating healthy meals? Do they contain all the proteins, minerals, and essential vitamins the body needs? If you did not know already, it is high time you knew what you are eating. The three meals of the day must be healthy and timely. If you are working in an office or are a salesperson, you will tend to order some fast food as and when you are hungry. This is a very unhealthy idea. Try and cook something healthy. If you cannot cook or have some recipes, you can do an online search. Many websites provide detailed recipes for vegetarian and non-vegetarian diets.

Salad with fruits and vegetables is a very healthy meal for people of all ages. It provides you with a lot of energy and keeps you fit. Doctors and nutritionists recommend a salad meal at least once a day. If you get tired of eating the same salad meal every day, you can add new flavours and bring in variety. You can also try different methods of preparing salads. Grilled, baked, and steamed food is always advisable.

A lot of people do not eat healthy because they cannot give up the foods they are used to and like. You can add items like boiled chicken, grilled pieces of steak, egg white and grilled bacon. This is primarily for people who do not wish to give up on steak and bacon. You can search online for healthy recipes that contain your favourite steak, bacon, ham, etc.

As much as possible, avoid eating fatty foods like egg yolk, bread, rice, and sugar. Eat brown and whole wheat bread, brown rice, and brown sugar instead. There are always healthy alternatives for every taste of food. In your meals, use ingredients that are sugar-free, cholesterol-free, and fat-free. This will help you remain fit and reduce risks to your cardiovascular system.

Know simple facts like:

   i.   Avoid using too much oil
  ii.   Do not overeat
 iii.   Use the right ingredients
 iv.   White and lean meats are better than fatty red meat
  v.   Dairy-based products are fattening
 vi.   Avoid deep-fried foods
vii.   Processed food is not all that great, though it might taste good
viii.   Junk food is filling but not healthy.
 ix.   Olive oil is the best cooking medium if at all you want to deep-fry something.
  x.   Instead of frying, stir-fry your vegetables.

Create time to search for food facts and what alternatives you can have. Learn ways to make meals with less fattening and yet healthy and tasty. Remember it is not only for you but your family also.

Your recipe should never contain a lot of non-vegetarian food, mainly if you are serving dinner because non-vegetarian food takes a bit longer to digest. Fruits and vegetables are always healthy options. Now that you have decided to eat healthy food, check the difference in your weight, skin, freshness and concentration in a few weeks and you will be pleasantly surprised at what you will discover.

Healthy Eating Plan for a Diabetic

If you are diabetic, you must be very careful of the foods you consume, as it is a malfunction where the body loses its control and overproduce insulin. The glucose level in the body fluctuates. A diabetic's diet plan must be different from the normal diet because many essential foods contain sugar, and these foods need elimination from a diabetic's diet. So, if you have diabetes, refer to a registered dietician or food counsellor.

Diet plan: Plan your diet. Note down all the foods you like eating. Separate the ones with sugar content. Doing this will enable you to know what you can consume, and at what rate. Your meal plan must include appropriate food and meal timings. You may ask your doctor or dietician for help in preparing this plan. Ensure that you check your blood pressure, blood sugar levels, and weight before you draw your meal plan. From the total calories consumed in a day, an average diabetic should target about 55% of carbohydrates, around 15% of proteins and 30% of fats.

Eating plan: Your eating plan should include edibles such as spinach, bitter gourd, and beets, as they are said to be low in glucose content. Fruits like gooseberry, blackberry, and oranges provide less glucose and more vitamins. It is advisable to eat about three times daily, in the recommended quantities. This is because people with diabetes, when very hungry, can faint. Eat more of green and leafy vegetables and use fat-free food products. Cut the drinking of alcohol, as it adds sugar to the body. If your sugar level is unstable, eat foods that contain adequate amounts of carbohydrates.

Here are some tips on how you can manage to reduce the level of sugar content in your body if you have diabetes.

- A glass of bitter gourd juice every morning can help you balance your sugar level. If you do not like the taste, you can have a glass of orange juice immediately after you drink it to change the taste of your mouth.

- Eat spinach, and tomatoes with your food.

- A glass of blackberry seed juice is considered a medicine for diabetics in many countries.

- Fenugreek seed juice is again suitable for people with diabetes.

If you carefully look, all the food mentioned above items are bitter or have no sugar content. Please consult your doctor or health counsellor before you try any of the tips mentioned above, as it might differ from person to person.

If your blood sugar level is high, you must completely stop the consumption of sugar and sweets and control the level of oil in your meals. Many people adhere to junk, oily, spicy and fattening food while managing their sugar levels. They may reduce the level of blood sugar but end up having heart problems. Therefore, it is essential to keep a check on your weight and blood pressure along with your sugar level. Eat healthy foods and reduce the risk of having diabetes.

Healthy Eating on a Budget

With food and fuel prices going through the roof, the world over, it has become imperative to restrict even necessary expenses and go on a budget. While it is essential to remain healthy, you can stay healthy on a budget.

It is not difficult when you know how. First, calculate the average monthly food expenses. Make sure you include everything from everyday expenses on vegetables, fruits, meat, and dairy products, and the money spent on going to restaurants bars. When you have the average amount of the past few months, it will become easy to plan your monthly budget. Since health is a priority, eliminate all the trips made to the local doughnut shop. You can still visit the doughnut shop but restrict it to twice or three times a month.

Substitute your doughnut break with fresh fruits or fruit or vegetable juices. If you want to eat something crunchy, make it a whole-wheat cracker or a couple of biscuits with a vegetable salad. The health benefits become visible almost immediately. The main savings come during your visit to the supermarket. Check your local newspapers and magazines for special offers and use food promo codes or coupons when available. Buy your vegetables and fruits in large quantities instead of buying them on a per-piece basis. It works out to be cheaper. Trimmed vegetables are also costly, so avoid them if you cannot afford them.

Most of the supermarkets have special schemes for juices and other canned items. Buy the ones that do not have preservatives or artificial colours and stick to the 100% natural ones instead. When buying meat products, avoid buying the boneless variety as they are costly. You can also remove the fat yourself from beef, instead of purchasing the more expensive low-fat variety.

Avoid eating red meat as much as possible and stick to white meat like chicken instead. It is good for your heart. Eat more vegetables with pasta, spaghetti, rice, etc., instead of overeating meat. Ensure to include potatoes, onions, garlic, ginger, and mint in your food. They are not only moderately cheap but also strengthen the immune system. When cooked with vegetables, they convert the dish into a tasty masterpiece.

You may need to modify your breakfast menu, and in case you eat high-fat and high-calorie foods such as fried bacon, eggs, and white bread, replace them with oatmeal, wholemeal bread, egg white, and whole wheat. You can make a smoothie by mixing bananas and strawberries in cold milk. It is low-cost yet satisfying. If you must eat bacon and egg, restrict yourself to eating it only once or twice a week. You may grill it instead of frying it.

Your dinner should also be light yet filling. Try to make pizzas and burgers at home. They are healthier and much cheaper compared to buying them from the restaurant. Instead of going to a bar regularly, invite a few friends home and enjoy your drinks with wholesome homemade foods together.

Instead of complaining about costly fuel and food prices over which you have no control, use it as an excuse to switch to healthier eating habits. Combine healthy eating with regular exercise to save money and live a long and healthy life.

CHAPTER THREE

Healthy Eating for All Ages

Many adults in America and Europe face obesity and other health-related problems. With changing lifestyles, adults ignore their nutritional needs. We eat either too much or too little. We are malnourished. Many of us lose the much-needed perfect balance of diet and proper eating habits in today's competitive world, where our attention is on greater earnings. This has affected us negatively and fill us with stress and mental pressures. It is high time we gave healthy eating a priority in our lives and spend our time living healthy.

Increasing life responsibilities requires us to consume more nutritious and healthy foods. With so much to do these days, the body should get all the essential minerals and vitamins as improper diets lead to body weakness, fatigue, and stress. Be cautious and have proper meals at the right time. Having little or improper food will not fulfil the body's needs, thereby making you sick and tired. This should be a good example and a warning to your children as you keep telling them to eat healthy to stay fit and live long.

Take note that junk food may reduce your hunger, but it does not take care of the body's nutritional needs. The body needs proteins and other essential vitamins and minerals to stay healthy. Junk food takes away vitamins from your body and instead adds extra saturated fats. This can lead to obesity which is an indicator of health problems. If you are not healthy, what can you do with your wealth? Unwholesome eating makes the body fall prey to health issues and you cannot enjoy life as you would keep feeling stressed and weak.

It is crucial to spare time to eat, and the time is now. Have small, but healthy meals at regular intervals. It does not matter whether you want to lose or add weight, you must eat breakfast every day. You will not lose weight by starving. Your body will only run short of the required amounts of nutrients. You may need to consult a nutritionist to help plan your daily diet, which you must follow if you want to live a healthy life. Proper food intake at appropriate times will keep you energetic all day long, and you can carry on with your activities without feeling stressed.

When you are well nourished, your brain gets sharp and more alert, and you perform well at work and home. You can manage life better than before. If they eat a proper diet, women will not need to buy expensive creams and lotions to get the glow on their face and body.

Keep eating healthy food and that radiance will stay with you always. Healthy food will invigorate your body system and help you to lead a healthy and active life. A good diet and adequate exercises keep diseases at bay. If the body gets what it needs, the immune system will become stronger and able to fight sicknesses and diseases. Even if you fall ill for any reason, your strong immune system will help you to recover faster.

It is not too late to appreciate the facts about healthy eating to healthy living. They go hand in hand. You can start with a good diet now and see the result for yourself. Therefore, the next time you walk into the market, do not forget to buy healthy foods for healthy eating.

Healthy Eating for Teenagers

Children need a lot of energy to perform their daily activities. An average teenager is involved in high-intensity activities every day compared to an office worker. Activities can be low, medium, and high intensity. Study, play, examinations, camping, excursions, big games, tours, are some of the activities that form part of a teenager's daily life. They need both mental and physical strengths with this routine to remain healthy and fit.

A teenager's meal should contain carbohydrates, proteins, minerals, and all the essential vitamins that their bodies need. A teenager should have more food as compared to a 45-year-old. This is because teenagers have high metabolism rates. Five to six medium meals justify an average teenager's food pattern. A little fatty food is not a problem because the fats in the body disappear the moment they start engaging in games, trips, or any other physical activities. Teenagers should eat heavy meals, as this is their only time to build healthy bodies. Healthy foods for teenagers include:

1. **Milk**

It provides calcium for healthy teeth and bones. Water content in the milk keeps you hydrated.

2. **Fruit juices**

These give the teenagers the boost in stamina required while they play.

3. Water

An average teenager must consume at least 8-10 litres of water per day.

4. Meat and eggs

Theyprovide proteins, vitamins, and carbohydrates. Very essential to increase weight and muscle mass. Fish helps in increasing concentration and alertness.

5. Fruits and vegetables

Theseare more essential than non-vegetarian food. It is essential because the minerals and vitamins are needed for the body and keep the body hydrated. Fruits also help in learning and remembering. Dieticians recommend plenty of fruits and vegetables for growing teens. Fruits and vegetables are an excellent option to gain weight and remain fit.

All these food items help teenagers in their studies and physical activities. A teenager should not eat too much oily or fattening foods, as this might make them lazy, sluggish, or even build excess body fats, which are the initial stages of obesity.

If your teenager is not engaged in sports or exercises, absolutely do not follow the foods mentioned above, since with healthy eating; there should always be good exercise. Teenagers with a low metabolism rate every so often put on more weight, even if they eat less. This is not correct.

The idea is to eat healthily and exercise more to increase the metabolism rate and reduce unwanted fats in the body.

Teenagers that are always on the computer or are at home should reduce the intake of meat, energy drinks, and milk, as these are not necessary for them and they might put on fats in their bodies. To conclude, teens should stop eating junk food from outside and stick to home-cooked food to stay healthy and fit.

Healthy Eating for People over Sixty

Generally, people over sixty have altered food tastes. Foods do not taste the same. They lose appetite, and even their favourite foods do not fascinate them anymore. They tend to put on weight even if they barely eat. Metabolism rates decrease with age, and people tend to put on fats. Increasing weight in the sixties is a bad sign, as it can cause many health-related hazards. A person in his or her sixties must follow a proper diet plan. Here are some tips on how you can maintain your weight and diet accordingly.

People usually do not work very hard in their sixties and therefore need less energy, but just enough to perform daily chores. Your diet must contain an adequate amount of protein, calcium, carbohydrates, and vitamins. Eat different varieties of food every day, so that it does not get monotonous and you have distinct taste every day. As you grow old, your bones tend to become weak and feeble. Your calcium level decreases, and you are likely to suffer from osteoporosis. To avoid these sufferings, you should drink enough low-fat milk and eat fat-free dairy products like cheese and butter. Make sure you do not gain fat.

Fruits and vegetables are a vital source of nutrition for persons of this age group, as they provide a sufficient amount of vitamins and minerals. Most fruits contain vitamins B and C. Vitamins, and calcium prevents memory loss and shivering. Protein in your diet must only be about 15-18% and mostly got from non-vegetarian foods like fish, eggs, and meat.

Always ensure that you keep your body well hydrated with water and juices. Water helps in cleansing the body from its impurities. Eat fibre-rich food like vegetables that provide proteins, too. More fibre in the body means fewer toxins. Fibre can be found in pulses and baked beans, prunes, and apricots. Do not eat a lot of sweet or sugar-based food because the empty calories present in them do not exactly provide energy but increases weight. Consumption of excess salt may raise high blood pressure, therefore, control intakes of salt and sugar.

Since senior people do not precisely engage themselves in physical activity, regular exercise, and a proper diet is a must. One has to increase metabolism rate, to remain fit and not put on excess weight. Older people often eat significantly less and cannot have three big meals. They should eat small meals at even intervals, which helps to increase their metabolism rate. Do not take any protein supplements or fats loss pills because they need vigorous workouts and are meant for people below 60.

Avoid tinned or packed food items, as they contain preservatives that are not healthy for persons of that age range. Some packaged foods also contain hydrogenated fats that may cause a problem in your cardio-vascular system. Eat proper amounts of food and ensure they are rich in nutrients so you can live a long and healthy life.

Healthy Eating for Infants

As a parent, you must take precautions about your infant's diet. The best food for an infant is breast milk. Usually, an infant is considered a baby of age 0 to 1 year old. People even think of preschoolers as infants. Let us categorize infants into different age groups and discuss their diet and precautions taken.

0 - 4 months: From the day of birth, until the infant is four months, there is no better food for the child than the mother's milk. Mother's milk contains all the essentials that a child needs in balanced amounts. The temperature, the thinness of the milk, germ-fighting and immunity enhancers, and many other factors ideal for the infant are present in the mother's breast milk. At this time, an infant is not ready to digest solid or semi-solid foods; therefore, continue breastfeeding until four to five months. Even if the baby gets diarrhoea, continue breastfeeding. It is best to continue breastfeeding the child up to the age of one year, but at this age, it is not possible.

5 - 6 months: You can now introduce your child to semi-solid food. At this age, the baby is not entirely ready to ingest semi-solid food but is partially all right. Feed your baby with cereals like wheat, maize or mashed fruits such as apples. Ensure you dilute the food with either the mother's breast milk or water. Feed the infant porridges. Feed the small infant amounts to time until it no longer is hungry. Do not force-feed your infant, as it might initially not eat and might throw up. This may happen because the infant is only used to sucking. The infant's food intake will gradually increase. Do not stop breastfeeding.

When your baby opens their mouth while feeding or their eyes follow the spoon, it means they are now ready to eat new food. Always feed your baby on your laps. This gives them a feeling of security.

7 - 9 months: After the baby gives a positive response to the semi-solid food, you can now bring in mild solid food. Small and fine pieces of fruits and vegetables, soft cheese, thin slices of chicken should be the child's meal. Initially, the child might not be delighted biting the food and might not eat. Therefore, it is advised not to stop breastfeeding. If your baby is hungry every two to four hours and wets the diapers four to six times a day, it means, your baby is getting food and fluids in the right quantity. Other indication could be the baby's weight increase.

10 - 12 months: The food in this period is not so different, but a little variation in the food is required. You can give bigger pieces of meat, fish, vegetables, and fruits. Cereals, mother's breast milk and fruit juices diluted with water are recommended as liquids. Always introduce new foods every two weeks. This can help you spot the foods that cause allergies or illness to your child. Maintain a high level of hygiene. Always boil water; always feed lukewarm food.

Healthy Eating During Pregnancy

Pregnancy is a time the woman's body needs more nutrition than before. As the development and growth of the fetus depend on what you eat, you must be careful with your eating habits. If the mother and the baby are deprived of vital proteins and minerals, there can be serious implications in the future. For a pregnant woman, it is important to stick to the doctor's advice and follow the diet that well suits the needs of a pregnant woman.

Do not be afraid of weight gain and eat less, and do not eat too much either. You can always work out and shed any extra weight. Do not skip meals. Eat heavy breakfast that may include cereal, fruit, milk, and other healthy foods. Eat in moderation. Eat more green vegetables, small portions of chicken, fish, beans, cheese, peanut butter, dried fruits, juices, soups, skimmed milk, and other dairy products. Every meal you eat should be rich in proteins, vitamins, and minerals. Avoid foods with allergic reactions.

If you have been a junk food addict, avoid it entirely as it can affect your baby. Eat what your body craves for. If you are a woman, being pregnant does not mean you should overeat. However, make sure there is not much gap in your meals and snacks, as your body will continuously need nutrition for the baby's growth. Be sensible when you choose food. Not eating responsibly when you are pregnant can cause your baby problems, and an underdeveloped baby is very difficult to take care of.

Being pregnant does not mean you should give up exercise. Exercising does not mean you must go to the gym and do your cardio or weights. Let there be some light exercises. Go on a walk or follow the activity that your doctor has asked you to follow. Being rigid and not moving around much can cause some difficulties at the time of delivery. So, it is important to allow your body to do some exercises as well. Be in the habit of taking a walk under fresh air so that you and your unborn baby get fresh oxygen to breathe.

Drink a lot of water and keep your body fully hydrated flushes out toxins from the body. Take liquids in the forms of soups and fruit juices. It is good to enjoy every of your meal and do not eat anything that may cause your baby discomfort. Certain foods can be a problem, so check with your doctor what to eat and what not to eat. Pregnancy is a susceptible period, and you need to be cautious enough to make sure you and your baby stay in good health.

Pregnancy is a time that you eat for two, so you need to be careful with your food choice. You must maintain a healthy diet all through your pregnancy, and even after the delivery, so you can recover much faster. Eating healthy will ensure the sound development of the baby, which is important for further growth.

Healthy Eating at Work

With increasing workplace stress and pressures at work, most employees hardly get time to think about their meals or to follow a health regimen. We know that to survive in this very competitive world, you have to go the extra mile to get noticed at your workplace. But that does not mean you have to compromise with your health. There are several ways to ensure your calorie and vitamin intake is sufficient for the day.

Firstly, it is essential to have breakfast before you leave home. This is the most important meal of the day, as it provides you with vigour for the whole day. For working women, it is very important to have milk for breakfast, and a combination of milk with oats or low-calorie cornflakes is ideal, as it is easy to make and provides you with calcium and the essential nutrients. If you have the time, you can also boil an egg and eat, as it will give you enough protein and cut out the carbohydrates.

While you are at work, you are bound to be tempted to have several cups of coffee but avoid this temptation. A cup of coffee a day may not be harmful, but once you start taking more than a cup a day, your calorie increases thereby resulting in body weight much faster.

You may have so much work in the office, you may be in a meeting, or you may be too consumed with work to realise you have skipped a meal or what you are eating is not very healthy. The first rule in healthy eating is to choose your food wisely. If you are in a meeting and you have been served a lunch, do not stuff your stomach with the cheese, pizzas, and sandwiches. Instead, go for salads or pizzas with green vegetable. Instead of a soft drink, take water or a fruit juice.

You can bring your food from home. Make a salad with a few chicken cubes and low-fat salad toppings for yourself. If you need bread, make sure it is brown. This type of meal is high in fibre and protein and helps you control or even lose weight.

After you get home, you tend to indulge in a snack, and so you tend to eat either fried or sweet food. Keep telling yourself that you have not indulged in any strenuous activity and you can always supplement your snacks with fruits or some refreshing juice.

Lastly, remember to have an early dinner rich in protein that includes meat and leafy vegetables to give you an ideal diet for the whole day. And very importantly, remember to get at least 20 minutes of exercise every day of the week to keep your body in good shape and stay fit.

CHAPTER FOUR

Feel Good and Look Young

Today's youth spend a lot on expensive creams and lotions to restore and maintain their beauty. The big question is: how many of them are successful in getting the glow on their face? If you do not eat a healthy diet, no cream will help you look young or feel good about yourself. You look what you eat, therefore, to look younger than your age and feel fresh and energetic throughout the day, take care of your eating habits.

If you meet any beautiful woman whose age looks the same for years together, make it a point, do ask them the secret behind it. They will tell you that the way to healthy skin and youthful looks are healthful foods, not any branded creams. To feel good and look young, change your diet. Being in the habit of eating healthy is the best solution for all your health problems. Consult a nutritionist for advice on the types of food you should eat. Due to their busy schedules, many people do not have the time to eat regular meals. However, food should be your priority, especially when you have a busy schedule. Kick-start your day with a heavy and nutritious breakfast, so you have enough energy throughout the day.

Cereals make a good breakfast. Replace white bread with brown bread and feel the difference. Drink a glass of juice or milk as per your choice. Add lots of leafy vegetables to your diet. Salads provide you with all the necessary vitamins. Some fruit after a meal is very healthy and enhances your energy levels. When shopping for meat, go for lean meat. This will keep a check on your fat levels. Fish is a good source of omega-3 fatty acids, and you should include fish in most of your meals. Beans, nuts, and eggs are high on proteins that the body requires for development. Do not completely cut down on fats as your body needs some for growth and development. You can choose low-fat foodstuffs to control your body fats.

A balanced diet makes sure you are high on energy levels and makes you feel lively all day long. Natural food items have all the minerals and essential vitamins that will make you feel good and look young. With healthy eating habits, you will not have to worry about any side effects or any health-related problems. Stay away from artificial juices and junk food. When in a restaurant, learn to select your dishes properly. It is good to order healthy and nutritious food. There is no reason to get bored with healthy food items, as you can experiment with your cooking. You can try various dishes and cook in different styles to make it look appetizing.

Eating Healthy When Dining Out

When you have started to eat healthy food at home, you need to extend it to dining out, since a single high-fat or high-calorie meal can spoil your entire week of healthy eating at home.

Narrow down restaurants that do not serve greasy or oily food or those that at least offers a healthier version of their regular food. You should inquire if the restaurant is willing to provide grilled or lightly sautéed dishes, instead of just frying them. Restaurants that serve different cuisines require different approaches.

But, as a rule of thumb, ensure that your consumption of fresh vegetables in the form of salads or other side dishes is high. The key to dining out is to savour the fine taste of various dishes. Instead of focusing on one item, try to eat small servings of various dishes. This will please your appetite while ensuring that you do not focus on a single high-calorie dish. Order a salad sprinkled with lime, salt, and pepper instead of one soaked with mayonnaise. When trying sauce-based meals, eat those that are tomato-based instead of cream-based. Avoid drinking sugared carbonated sodas, and instead, drink tea or coffee, or better still drink fresh fruit juices or water.

Avoid soups that have a lot of cream content and instead stick to clear soup or tomato soup. A soup will dull your appetite, and so, you will not overeat. Try not to finish the whole dish at once, but instead get some of it packed to warm the next day.

www.ingramcontent.com/pod-product-compliance
Lightning Source LLC
Chambersburg PA
CBHW070105260726
48658CB00002B/996